ISBN-13:
ISBN-10:

Cover design by: Art Painter
Library of Congress Control Number:
Printed in the United States of America

CONTENTS

MEAL PREP
FOR BEGINNERS

INTRODUCTION

What is meal prepping? Meal prep is to prepare most of your meals ahead of time; you plan what you are going to take for a week or, even more, a month. You cook all the meals yourself, ensuring that you have a healthier and unprocessed meal on the table.

Meal prepping helps us focus on our daily nutrition, leading to improved health and reducing the unwanted fats in our bodies. When this is priority number one, healthier habits will develop, and you will find your life turning around and becoming much more confident.

To start with, it's important to plan what meals you are going to cook. It will really help if you start out with a small time-frame for two or three days, then proceed to weeks and months. You should start simple and not complicate things trying to prepare the most elaborate, fanciest meals around. For a newbie, it is crucial to start small and simple. Keep it straight-forward and healthy, that's the primary concern here. Once you have your plan in hand, you can then make your grocery list, so you will have everything needed to prepare all those meals. Remember, you will find some healthy recipes later in the book that will help you kick-start the journey to meal prepping.

You will also learn that cooking extra portions is one of the best tips you should get in the habit of doing when it comes to meal prepping. For instance, if you are planning to cook Paleo orange chicken for dinner, simply cook a couple of extra portions and you will then have the perfect meal for next week's dinner. You can always freeze the meal and enjoy later on in the week to come. Having snacks already portioned and stored will increase the likelihood of your family members maintaining their healthy eating.

A freezer will be an important piece of equipment when it comes to meal prepping. Get in the habit of storing meals that are already appropriately portioned into containers and label with the date, so you know when it was prepared. You can do the same thing with snacks too. When you purchase fruit and veggies from the market, cut them into snack-sized bites and portion them into baggies or containers. Label and place in the freezer if you aren't planning on eating them in the next few days. We will learn more about storage, types of equipment needed, healthy cooking tips, etc. later on in the book.

Meal prepping comes with a lot of advantages; you will be able to plan your meals for the upcoming days/week, lessen the trips to fast food spots, and at the same time keep everyone eating in a more healthy manner. Here's the perfect opportunity to start developing a healthy eating plan to keep you focused on nutrition and appropriate portion sizes, which in turn will lead to weight loss and a stronger commitment to maintaining a healthy life.

CHAPTER 1

WHY SHOULD I MEAL PREP?

Apart from living healthier and losing weight, there are other reasons why everyone should meal prep now and then. Here are some extra tips on why everyone should consider doing it, at least some of the time:

- Saves money - One of the top reasons to start meal prepping is that you will save money. That's because you're able to buy more foods in bulk. Consider how much you would save by purchasing your meat and veggies in bulk, instead of just buying small portions that you need for one or two meals. You can then prep your meals and gain all of the other benefits as well. Plus you save money by not making as many different meals and by avoiding eating out.

- Saves time - If you're someone who often skips making home cooked meals during the week because you don't have lot of time due to work and other responsibilities, meal prepping will be perfect for you. Choose an evening or weekend when you have some extra time and prepare or cook most of the meals for the week. That way, all that needs to be done is to put your meals together and do some minor heating up or cooking the rest of the days of the week.

- Eat healthier - Meal prepping ensures that you will eat healthier meals since every single meal is very carefully planned out. You'll be making multiple healthy meals at one time, often using fresh or frozen produce, lean protein, and other natural ingredients. It also helps you to learn portion control. Use meal prep containers that include compartments that separate different parts of the meals into proper portion sizes.

- Stay committed to your diet - Since you will have all your meals for the entire week prepped up, packed, and ready to eat, you know in advance that you will always be on track when it comes to your nutrition goals. You can plan your meals with the goal of losing weight. You can plan your meals ahead of time so that you will eat enough food and take in enough calories for a healthy weight gain.

- You get to regulate your portion intake and size - Have you taken the time to notice just how large the portion sizes are when you order fast food? Do you know how many calories you're getting from each meal served? When you meal prep, you control the number of calories in each portion or each meal. You know how much protein you're getting. You know how much fat and carbs you're getting.

HOW MEAL PREPPING SUPPORTS WEIGHT LOSS

Meal prepping will help you lose the excess weight when planned right. Meal prepping will always have an impact on how you look and feel. If you work-out but eat unhealthy foods and forget the essential nutrients your body needs to reduce the excess fats, you're only working your way towards failure. By picking the right recipes and ingredients, you will find that meal prep is a lifestyle change that is viable long term. You may not see dramatic and fast results; however, there is a much greater chance that your weight loss will be sustainable using these techniques.

Meal prepping helps you to be more aware of how many calories you consume as opposed to eating unhealthy food on the go. It also contributes to ensuring that you are consuming the right nutrients, vitamins, and minerals necessary to sustain a healthy diet. By planning out your meals in advance and around your life demands, you can make smart choices much more quickly. Prepping meals that consist of low fat, low sodium, or non-processed ingredients significantly surpasses any options at fast food restaurants. It is this combination of nutritional downfalls that make fast food an enemy to the progression of your health and fitness goals.

It is paramount that you take a look at your eating habits and what triggers are causing you to make poorer choices. There are chemicals in processed foods that your body can become dependent on or even addicted to that are commonly found in the foods served in fast food restaurants. That is why people get cravings for fast food, or why people feel that only a cold soda will quench that thirst. Avoid that temptation and don't give in to the cravings by not giving yourself the opportunity to have them. Have ready to go meals prepared for your busy lifestyle by cooking your food in advance.

It takes a strong sense of dedication and willpower to eat right when you are trying to lose weight and get in shape. Don't be hard on yourself when you slip up, but work hard to always stay on track. By meal prepping, you can continue to see the progress that you want because you are eating the healthy foods that your body needs and desires while cutting out the ones that set you back. You should particularly note your calorie intake, excess calories in our bodies leads to fat storage.

However, calories provide our bodies with energy. Let's learn a little bit about how they are useful for our bodies when taken in the required amount. Calories is a measurement of energy; it is the unit that energy in the body is measured in. Our bodies need energy to work, so as much as we hate them, we physically need calories to live. Our beating hearts needs calories. Our brains need calories. The problem is when we have too many calories and our bodies store them for later use as fat. The 'later', however, often never comes and the calorie storage and our waistline grow.

The number of calories we should eat per day are based on our age, sex, and activity level. Women, in general, need fewer calories than men. For us to lose weight, our daily calorie needs (what our body uses) must be higher than the calories we take in. This forces the body to resort to the stored energy to continue to function. If our metabolism thinks we're eating too little, it will put us into starvation mode. Starvation mode is when your body lowers your metabolic rate and packs every extra calorie into body fat.

CHAPTER 2

HOW TO HAVE A HEALTHY LIFESTYLE

What you take into your stomach will reflect how healthy you will be in future. Developing good eating habits will lead to a healthy way of life. You should watch what you eat and ensure that it is beneficial to your health. The best way to adjust to healthy eating habits is to reflect on the bad eating habits you were used to and replace them with good and healthy eating habits. Having a healthy lifestyle starts in your mind and moves down to executing those actions. It may sound difficult from the word go, but you have to keep on reinforcing the healthy eating habits until they become a part of you.

You need to make some changes in your life to bring about the desired progress towards your healthy eating goals. Some of these promising changes include:

Water - The effect of water in a healthy lifestyle is that it not only provides vital hydration, but it's also a zero calorie drink, meaning you're burning more calories to consume it than in the liquid itself. By drinking water first, you can often assuage your hunger without eating. It is ideal for cutting your calorie intake. After taking your breakfast, the rest of the day just make water your primary drink. This keeps your cravings in control and ensures that you do not overeat.

Avoid soft drinks, which are high in calories due to the added sugars. Sugary drinks trigger your cravings and only make you want you to eat. This makes you overeat and hence more calories for your body to turn and store as fat.

Fruits And Vegetables - Most people have embraced the thought of eating from fast foods stores and ordering food to be brought to their doorstep as the right way. This is very wrong and is the main reason for the rise in overweight people and obesity across the globe. There has also been immense consumption of processed foods in many homes starting from corn flakes during breakfast to t.v. meals at dinner time. These foods are hazardous and result in accumulation of unwanted fat in the body, especially around the abdominal area. Processed and fast foods are not well balanced in terms of essential nutrients as compared to fruits and vegetables. In fact, they are packed with excess calories that are harmful to bodily health, and worse, make you add unnecessary weight.

The best solution is to adopt a lifestyle of having fruits and vegetables as much as you can in each meal of the day. The fruits and vegetables are of great value to your body's health and weight. You have witnessed how healthy vegans are in terms of weight. This is because the fruits and vegetables contain essential ingredients that are readily broken down and absorbed by the body's enzymes. In fact, some of the components in fruits and vegetables replenish the body's cells and ensure that they work optimally. On the other hand, the fast and processed foods are full of unbalanced ingredients with a proportion of them being harmful to the body's cells. These foods are full of fats and calories that make you add unnecessary weight and some of the harmful ingredients like bad LDL cholesterol result in heart problems and cancer development.

Eat Healthy Unprocessed Food - There has been an increase in the consumption of processed and packaged foods over the years. This is a dangerous trend and is one of the reasons for the increase in obesity and overweight cases. The problem is that the packaged foods do not contain balanced nutrients. They are high in fat, salt sugar and lack essential nutrients and fiber. You should develop the habit of preparing meals from unprocessed foods, which unlike processed foods are high in essential nutrients and fiber. Unprocessed foods are low in calories and have soluble monosaturated fats, which are easily broken down by the body.

Eat Healthy Portion Sizes - The body requires a small percentage of what we eat for its optimal cell metabolism. The rest of the food ingredients is eliminated as waste or stored as fat for later use. The more food you eat, the more excess calories and sugars. The excess sugars are converted and stored in the body as fat, especially around the belly.

You are just supposed to eat a small portion of food with all the essential nutrients for your body's growth and development. You should avoid taking large food portions, rather divide your meals so that you can have small portions of food a maximum of five times a day. It is important that you cut your meal proportions to smaller sizes and instead have healthy snacks in between breakfast, lunch, and dinner. This helps you to consume less, and you never get hungry and so have your cravings in check. You can choose to have fruits as your snacks, but make sure the foods are low in calories and within the allowed daily calorie limit.

Salads and Soups - By selecting a soup and salad option, you're often taking a higher fiber and more nutrient dense meal. The fiber in the food will not only curb your appetite, but it will take more time to be digested, and you'll feel fuller longer. Foods like this tend to be much lower in calories or require much larger portions to make up the same calorie amount.

CHAPTER 3
HOW TO GET STARTED

While it will take practice to build a routine, there are ways that you can set yourself up for success from the outset.

Write Down Your Plan - While it may sound tedious or too simple, taking the time to document each meal forces you to think through your meal prep strategy. It also forces you to consider every ingredient that you will need before cooking so that you don't start cooking and realize halfway through that you are out of cinnamon or ginger. Consider writing out your plan on a calendar so that you have each day and meal planned out precisely.

Make Time - Meal prepping is something that you need to take the time to do right. It is your chance to be dedicated to your health and fitness goals, and it isn't something to skimp out on or take lightly. Make sure you set aside a couple of hours to do your meal prepping properly. It includes everything from planning, shopping, prepping the food, and then cooking it. Rushing through the process could leave room for errors and then lead to wasted food, time, and money.

Many people allocate a day of the week to cook in bulk. Being consistent will help you to form a habit and commit to the process. Try starting with a few days' worth of meals at a time, then slowly building up to making a whole week of meals in one session.

Don't Stray from Your Grocery List - Making a grocery list

after you have structured your meal plan and determined the ingredients you need is essential to successful prepping. When you head to the grocery store, don't do it without a list in hand. Whether you write down your list or store it on your phone, the list is going to keep you on track with the healthy food choices that you planned out. There are also plenty of apps that you can download onto your phone to make it easier to keep track of what you need. Straying sets you up to either forget a necessary ingredient and need to take a trip to the store a second time, or it will cause you to purchase items that you don't need, and you can end up wasting that food or adding those calories to your waistline.

Go for Different Recipes Each Day - If you eat the same food every day, you will quickly tire of that meal and seek out cheat options. Ensure you diversify and mix up your recipes so that you won't be put off by the thought of the same dinner for the fourth night in a row. Rotate your recipes frequently and as you get more comfortable with different meals, try to make some of the cuff alterations to some of your tried and true favorites.

Make It a Social Thing - Why meal prep alone? Meal prepping and then doing swaps with your friends is a great way to try out new things and overcome monotony. Each of you can cook additional portions of one meal in bulk before exchanging portions. It allows you to save even more time by focusing on one meal (less shopping and cooking), but being able to consume two or more differing recipes. The best part is that you will end up creating a community of healthy minded people who will support each other along their health and fitness journeys.

Stretch Your Ingredients - When picking recipes for meal prep, try to group them by overlapping or common ingredients. For example, eggs with peppers and onions make a great breakfast, and you can use more of the peppers and onions to make fajitas for dinner that night. It will make your shopping easier as well and potentially cut down on costs. To help with switching up your meal planning so that you don't get sick of the recipes, alternate those ingredients that you use as a staple one week to another food the next.

Bake Your Food All at Once - If you are roasting vegetables, prepping sweet potatoes, and baking chicken, it is possible to knock out cooking all of those foods at once in your oven. Each of those meals prepared separately would mean that you are spending multiple hours waiting for each batch to be done. By combining them in the oven on multiple racks, you can save time in your meal prep and use less gas or electricity in the process. Prep all of your food that you want to bake in the oven on individual baking sheets and set the oven to a temperature that works best for all of them.

Keep a close eye on ingredients that might cook faster than others so that they don't burn. Likewise, make sure you keep a meat thermometer handy so that you don't take your proteins out before they are cooked all the way through. Ensure that you use separate chopping boards and utensils where appropriate to avoid cross contamination of raw foods.

Prep Your Proteins - An easy way to meal prep and have your food ready to go for the week is to prepare mostly a mini buffet or salad bar in your fridge. By utilizing well-organized storage containers, grab and create your meals with all of the ingredients that you want. To help with this approach, it is essential that you cook your proteins such as chicken, pork, ground turkey, etc. in advance. As a general rule, most cooked meats will last for three to four days in the refrigerator. It makes it easy to grab the protein that you want and add them to a quinoa bowl, wrap, or salad to round out a well-balanced meal.

CHAPTER 4

HOW TO PREPARE AND COOK FASTER

In this crazy world with busy lifestyles, we have found ourselves neglecting taking time and preparing nice healthy meals for our bodies. You may busy at your workplace, but I will help you prep your meals faster so that you are always consuming the right, healthy foods within a short period. If you work hard at it, you can become efficient at meal prepping and complement a full schedule. I will outline some of the techniques to help speed up your cooking:

Bake in Large Quantities - This is a speed prepping technique that makes all of the difference, particularly for lunch box or breakfast staples. Baking your food in bulk really helps to cut down on the amount of time spent on snack sized items. For example, if you are making your breakfast food for the week, you can bake eggs with meat and vegetables in muffin tins for a high protein and filling meal. You can store the individual muffins in containers or ziplock bags and just grab the portion you need for the day, reheat it, and be out the door in a flash, or cook a loaf of banana bread and portion into wrapped slices to have with afternoon tea. I know this method has saved me quite a few dollars over time that would otherwise have gone to the work cafe.

Utilize the Pressure Cooker Meals – Make use of your pressure cooker to meal prep as it takes a fraction of the time and energy compared to conventional methods, while not compromising on flavor. Most foods cook much faster than they usually would when using this approach, in many cases up to one-third faster. Pressure cookers are also a healthy way to prepare meals as less oil is typically used, while vitamins and minerals are better preserved due to shortened heat exposure. Curries, hearty beef stews, and risottos are just a small assortment of family favorites that can be made in this handy appliance.

One-Pot Meals - If you want to prepare tasty meals which still provide extended nutritional benefits, try one-pot cooking for ease of cleanup and simplicity. Note that the "one-pot" can also refer to one baking tray, skillet, or steamer depending on your recipe. There are plenty of delicious options online, and this method lends itself to the use of extra food scraps or leftover meat cuttings. Although some recipes may not allow for the perfect balance of protein, carb, and vegetable, this can be remedied by adding prepped food such as quinoa or rice that you have made for the week. Another benefit of this technique is saving power and gas usage, and most importantly, less dish washing!

Master Mixes - This process refers to part assembling or cooking some components of your recipes. These can be stored in the fridge or freezer to give you a head start on meals. For example, pre-season your ground meats into portioned bags for use in future recipes such as tacos and pasta sauces. Another idea is to prep your protein at once by seasoning chicken and baking it in one pan, but separate out the different flavors that you want to use.

You can also cut up your vegetables into quick stir fry bags along with some onions and minced garlic. Note that some vegetables require blanching before being frozen. Do this to avoid mushy and flavorless beans, broccoli, and other veggies such as asparagus. There are many home delivery food services which also do this and send you a box of raw vegetables and cooked proteins for compiling.

Freeze the Servings Once Cooled - Then when you are ready to eat it just defrost in the microwave and then reheat until steaming. If you want to go one further, soaking the grains overnight with a dash of vinegar or lemon juice (makes the nutrients in grains more digestible and more easily assimilated by our bodies) will halve your cooking time.

Bag Your Smoothies - Smoothies make a great breakfast on the go or a fulfilling recovery for your post workout. Don't waste your time during the week grabbing various ingredients out of the fridge and making your smoothie one ingredient at a time. You can prepare your smoothies in advance and store them in frozen portioned bags until you are ready to enjoy. Distribute your preferred serving of fruits, kale, spinach, or whatever else you want to have in your smoothie into a line up of zip lock bags. When you are ready to drink your smoothie, simply empty the bag contents into your blender, add in liquids such as water, almond milk, yogurt, coconut water, or protein powder, and blend away for a quick fix.

Pre-Assemble Your Salads - Salads are a staple of a healthy diet because they are comprised mainly of non processed ingredients. Save valuable time during the week by creating them in advance. Try putting them in mason jars for quick, grab and go meals during the week. To avoid getting your greens soggy, ensure that you start with placing any dressing on the bottom (or in a separate small container) followed by hard vegetables, any grains or beans, cheeses, softer vegetables and then your leafy mix. Add proteins such as chicken or hard boiled eggs on the day you plan to eat the salad.

MEAL PREPPING HACKS AND IDEAS

Below, you will all get to know all the best ideas that will help the meal prepping process become easier, faster, and simpler. The ideas will make sure your meal plan is healthier than you could imagine.

Start Simple and Small - Meal prepping should make things easy and the recipes should be easy. If you're just starting or if you have some experience at meal prepping, then stick to simple dishes and recipes. You may not have time to prepare and preserve an elaborate dinner or lunch. You can do your master chef wizardry on the day when you assemble your meals for eating.

You can start by prepping just trail mix, eggs, snacks, and veggies at first. Once you have gotten used to preparing small meals and snacks, then it's time to try breakfasts. After that add lunches and dinners. Eventually, you reduce the times you buy your meals from restaurants. Finally, you have all your meals prepped and ready. Take things one step at a time until you are so used to the drill you can do things with an arm and a leg tied behind your back.

Try To Get Larger Cooking Devices - Get larger pots, larger baking pans, a larger grill if you want to cook big food portions at once.

Invest in Good Meal Prepping Containers - You will need a place to store all the food you're preparing, and nothing is better than Tupperware. Be sure it can go from the fridge to the microwave to the freezer without an issue.

Use Your Slow Cooker - Using a slow cooker is by far the most straightforward and basic way to make healthy eating easy.

Fruits - Nothing is easier than smearing a little nut butter on a banana or apple. They are a very healthy and relatively low-calorie fruit to include in your eating plan.

Pick the Food Product on Your Food List - Shopping around the grocery store will be much faster if you already have a bunch of foods on your list. It can be anything from chicken, potatoes, greens, shrimp, oatmeal, apples, etc. You already know what to look for, and you have an idea where to find them.

Choose the Right Containers from the Get-Go - Glass food containers, like mason jars, tend to last longer than plastic food boxes. You can say that it is an investment. Quality containers will allow you to portion your meals easily. Choose containers of different shapes and sizes. Some will be used for salads and others for snacks. Larger ones will be for lunches and dinners.

Your Lids Should Match - It will be quite frustrating getting the wrong lids for your containers. You don't have time to match the lids. It would be great if you can find containers that have the same lids so you can use one or the other, especially when they're reusable, and you have washed them well.

Keep Looking for New Recipes - Since you don't want your meals to be boring – they will get boring after you have cooked them and stored for about a week or two – look for the next interesting and healthy recipe you find.

Keep the Shopping List Detailed - You can use any note taking app on your phone and make sure that you keep your list detailed. You can also add notes of your inventory. It doesn't matter if it's just chopped garlic or cuts of lean meat. The important thing is that you have an idea of every detail of your pantry.

Make Your Meals Pretty - Since you're in the business of cooking your food, try to be creative and get them looking beautiful. Food tastes better if you can make it look tempting. Looking at the same thing over and over again isn't going to be that appealing, especially if you've seen it a hundred times.

Use a Timer - Meal prepping can seem quite overwhelming. However, if you create blocks of time, you can breeze through each task and get things done before you know it. A timer will help you track how long you have been working on something. It will also prompt you to get the tray out of the oven before everything gets burned. Some people enjoy preparing meals so much they use up their entire Sunday just for it. You should know when to stop and enjoy the rest of your day.

Pre-Cut Corners - One way to save on time is to buy pre-cut veggies and other produce. That way you don't have to spend so much time chopping and dicing. You get more time to do a lot of other stuff, and you can get your meal prep done a lot easier.

Get Containers that are Functional - Find containers that are easy to stack and are dishwasher safe. If you can find containers that you can arrange and stack easily with other containers, then get those.

Double the Volume of Your Purchases - Examine your grocery list. Double big items on that list like produce, proteins, fats, etc. Increasing the amount of stuff for these items means that you can cook them once and then eat them on several days of the week.

CHAPTER 6

PROPER LONG-TERM FOOD STORAGE TIPS

TIPS ON HOW TO STORE FOODS FOR LATER USE

Since we are going to cook some food in large quantities for later use, it is necessary to develop proper food storage practices. Food storage is an essential factor to consider when it comes to meal prepping. Here are some food storage tips which will help to retain flavor quality without compromising the safety of consumption.

Wrap Your Food Carefully - Wrapping your food carefully is key to preservation. To keep freezer burn (when air dries out the surface of foods, toughening the texture and worsening flavors) away from your meats and other foods, ensure you wrap and seal your food so that no part is exposed. If you do not seal or contain items carefully, you will allow space for air to get in and that can spoil certain items.

Label Your Items - You should try to mark each item with the item or meal name along with the date. Use a sharpie or dry erase marker for this depending on the surface. Go one step further and use different colored markers for cooked and raw items. You should always know how long food has been in the freezer.

Store Small, Manageable Food Portions - You should not make one big recipe and store it all in the biggest container you can find. It is not efficient and will waste valuable ingredients. To combat this, you need to portion out individual servings of your recipes.

It makes it much easier when you defrost food because you are not taking more out of the freezer than you need at that moment. Food safety risk is not in the freezing, rather, it is in the thawing process. Use smaller portioned sized containers to manage this. Do not fill your jars and containers to capacity to avoid messy overflow or explosions.

Arrange the Items in the Freezer Accordingly - Even though you may have prepped meals and frozen leftovers with the best of intentions, often these remnants are shoved to the back of the freezer and long forgotten. Allocate specific shelves or areas of your freezer rather than random placement for meals which need to be consumed. Some labels which could be used include "cooked meals", "uncooked proteins/meat", and "stock or dump meal scraps." It also goes for frozen ingredients which are yet to be utilized in your recipes. Ensuring that they are visible will result in less wastage at the end of the day if you plan wisely.

Optimize Freezer Storage - When storing individual servings of food items such as berries or pancakes, spread them onto a tray and freeze first in a single layer. Once they have frozen, they will not stick together, and you can place them all in a compact bag. For liquid items such as stocks and soups, allow them to cool and then pour into a plastic zip lock bag placed horizontally. It enables them to be stackable once frozen as opposed to having multiple jars of differing shapes.

THE FREEZER BASICS TIPS

Regarding temperature, your refrigerator should be 38 - 40°F and your freezer should be set to at least 32°F (0°C) or below. This range ensures that the variety of food items are unlikely to form bacteria and stay fresh for longer. If your fridge doesn't have a digital thermometer, then it's worth investing in a small portable one. Be quick when opening up your freezer door. It takes up to half an hour for the freezer temperature to chill down again after each use.

Efficient Freezer Use - Freezers run more efficiently when full. Use tubs of ice cream, bread loaves, or meal packs to reduce gaps. Concerning placement, ensure that your freezer is positioned correctly with space at the back for air to circulate efficiently. Don't sit the freezer next to a sunny window or against a hot cooktop. Clean the dust away from the freezer coils at the back on a quarterly basis. It helps to reduce the energy consumption.

Freezing Procedures - Whenever you are freezing your food, you need to make sure that you give the food enough time to cool down before you put it in a container to freeze. Freezing food when hot will only increase the temperature of the freezer and could cause other foods to start defrosting. Additionally, when you are putting anything in a bag, squeeze out any extra air to avoid freezer burn. When you are taking out food to thaw, reheat it thoroughly and do not refreeze to be extra safe. Further to this, add no more than 20 percent of the freezer capacity of unfrozen foods at one time. Set the freezer to fast freeze so that it is extra cold and add new items in batches.

NOVICE MEAL PREPPING MISTAKES TO AVOID

- Don't Eat While Meal Prepping – Avoid eating any snack while you prep to avoid undermining the entire point of meal prep. To ensure you're not overeating during prep time, keep yourself busy or chew gum.

- Packing The Same Meal Every Day - While it's easier than dreaming up new meal options for every day, chances are you'll get burnt out on the same grilled chicken on top of a spinach salad for lunch daily.

- Not Cooking At The Right Time – Make sure to follow a certain routine to avoid inconsistency. For instance, when you start on Sunday, which of course is the most commonly preferred day to start with, it will allow you to have an incentive to cook because you want to start the next week on the right foot and also most people have Sunday off, and they are relaxed and not under any time pressure to get anything else done.

- Shortage of Food Supplies – Make sure you buy the ingredients for a variety of possible meals, so you'll feel satisfied every time you eat.

CHAPTER 5
44. HEALTHY RECIPES

In this chapter, you will get to know where to outline some of the best recipes that will help you kick-start the meal prep journey. You will find breakfast, lunch, dinner, and dessert recipes. With these kind of recipes, you will lose the excess fat in your body and get back in shape soon.

BREAKFAST RECIPES

1. TASTY POPEYE PIE

Serves: 6

Prep Time: 20 minutes

Cooking Time: 35 minutes

INGREDIENTS:

- 4 slices paleo-approved bacon, diced
- 45 ml (3 tablespoons) almond milk
- 6 eggs, whisked
- 1 red onion, chopped
- 1 cooked sweet potato, mashed
- 1 tomato, deseeded and chopped
- 15 ml (1 tablespoon) of jalapeños pepper finely minced or 5 ml of crushed dried chilies
- 1 bag of baby leaves spinach, grossly shopped
- 15 ml (1 tablespoon) flat leaf parsley, Italian parsley
- Sea salt and freshly ground pepper to taste

INSTRUCTIONS:

1) Preheat oven to 180ºC/350°F.

2) Lightly grease a baking pie dish with olive oil spray.

3) Combine well all ingredients in a mixing bowl. Season with salt and pepper.

4) Place batter into the pie dish.

5) Bake for 30 to 35 minutes or till golden browned.

Nutritional Information (per serving)

Calories: 330

Fat total: 24.3g

Saturated fat: 15.2g

Carbohydrates: 15.9g

Dietary fiber: 2.8g

Sugars: 6.0g

Protein: 13.6g

2. DELICIOUS PUMPKIN BREAKFAST PANCAKES

Prep Time: 5 minutes

Cooking Time: 10 minutes

INGREDIENTS:

- 30 ml (2 teaspoons) coconut oil
- 250 ml (1 cup) pumpkin, pre-boiled and mashed
- 15 ml (1 tablespoon) almond butter
- 5 ml (1 teaspoon) pumpkin pie spice
- 5 ml (1 teaspoon) cinnamon
- 5 ml (1 teaspoon) vanilla extract
- 2 eggs, lightly beaten
- 1 tablespoon toasted almonds, chopped
- 15 ml (1 tablespoon) maple syrup

INSTRUCTIONS:

1) Mash pumpkin in a bowl. Mix with almond butter.

2) Add in pumpkin pie spice, cinnamon, and vanilla extract and mix well.

3) Stir in eggs and whisk to combine well.

4) Heat oil in a nonstick skillet on medium heat.

5) Add 3 heaping tablespoons of batter into the pan and cook pancake for 2-3 minutes or until nicely golden. Flip and cook the other side and repeat until all batter is gone.

6) Serve on a plate, sprinkled with toasted nuts and drizzled with maple syrup.

Nutritional Information (per serving)

Calories: 258

Fat total: 16.1g

Saturated fat: 6.2g

Carbohydrates: 21.2g

Dietary fiber: 5.0g

Sugars: 10.9g

Protein: 9.4g

3. SWEET PALEO APPLE AND SPICE MUFFINS

Serving: 12

Prep time: 15 minutes

Cooking time: [1]

INGREDIENTS

- 2 cups almond flour
- 2 teaspoons baking powder
- 3 apples (peeled and shredded)
- 2 tablespoons maple syrup
- ¾ cup coconut milk
- 2 large eggs
- 2 tablespoons coconut oil
- 1 teaspoon cinnamon
- 1/8 teaspoon nutmeg
- Vegetable cooking spray

INSTRUCTIONS:

1) Preheat your oven to 180ºC/350°F. Grease muffin tin with cooking spray. In a bowl, mix dry ingredients together well.

2)   In another bowl, mix all wet ingredients until well combined. Add the mixture to the dry ingredients and whisk well.

3) Add the minced apple to the batter and mix well. Pour the batter into each muffin hole until they are 3/4 full.

4)   Bake for around 18-20 minutes until cooked thoroughly. You can check by inserting a toothpick in the middle of one of the muffins.

Nutrition Information (per muffin)

Calories: 168

Carbs: 17 g

Fat: 5.5 g

Protein: 3 g

Sugars: 16.3g

4. LITTLE BLACK DRESS OMELET

Serves: 4

Prep Time: 10 minutes

Cooking Time: 10 minutes

INGREDIENTS:

- 250 ml (1 cup) onion
- 250 ml (1 cup) spinach
- 1 tomato (sliced)
- 30 ml (2 tablespoons) coconut oil
- 8 egg whites
- Sea salt and freshly ground pepper to taste
- Tomato and cucumber slices for garnish

INSTRUCTIONS:

1) Heat the oil in a large skillet, cook onions for 2-3 minutes until fragrant and tender. Add the tomatoes and spinach and sauté for another 2-3 minutes.

2) Add egg whites to the vegetables. Season with salt and pepper to taste. Cook for 2-3 minutes until the sides become golden brown and the omelet is fully cooked.

3) Fold half the omelet on the other side.

4) Serve with tomato and cucumber slices.

Nutritional Information (per serving)

Calories: 160

Fat total: 13.8g

Saturated fat: 11.8g

Carbohydrates: 4.4g

Dietary fiber: 1.1g

Sugars: 2.3g

Protein: 6.2g

5. SWEET, ALL DAY PANCAKES

Serves: 4

Prep Time: 10 minutes

Cooking Time: 15 minutes

INGREDIENTS:

- 6 eggs, lightly beaten
- 250 ml (1 cup) almond milk
- 250 ml (1 cup) almond flour
- 125 ml (½ cup) coconut flour
- 60 ml (¼ cup) ground flaxseed
- 1 medium-sized, very ripe banana, mashed
- 30 ml (2 tablespoon) maple syrup
- 5 ml (1 teaspoon) vanilla
- 5 ml (1 teaspoon) apple cider vinegar
- 1 ml (¼ teaspoon) sea salt
- 30 ml (2 tablespoons) of coconut butter
- Maple syrup, to drizzle or fresh fruits with raw honey

INSTRUCTIONS:

1) Combine eggs, mashed banana, almond milk, maple syrup,

vanilla, and vinegar in a large mixing bowl. Beat for 2-3 minutes until light and fluffy.

2) Mix all the dry ingredients in a bowl. Add gradually to the egg mixture and blend well, beating at low speed for 2-3 minutes. You can also use a food processor and blend all ingredients for 1-2 minutes on medium speed.

3) Heat a large non-stick frying pan and melt the coconut butter. Spoon about 60 ml (1/4 cup) of this batter into the pan and cook for 2-3 minutes or until slightly golden. Flip and cook other side. Repeat until all batter is gone.

4) Sprinkle pancakes with maple syrup or fresh fruits with some raw honey.

Nutritional Information (per serving)

Calories: 311

Fat total: 24.6g

Saturated fat: 8.5g

Carbohydrates: 14.2g

Dietary fiber: 3.3g

Sugars: 7.2g

Protein: 11.2g

6. TASTY CAVEMAN HASH

Serves: 4

Prep Time: 15 minutes

Cooking Time: 25 minutes

INGREDIENTS:

For the sausage patties:

- 450 g (1 pound) of ground pork or veal
- 1-2 garlic cloves, minced
- 2 1/2 ml (½ teaspoon) jalapeños, minced, or 1 ml (¼ teaspoon) crushed hot chilies flakes
- 2 1/2 ml (½ teaspoon) dry thyme
- 2 1/2 ml (½ teaspoon) dry rosemary
- 1 ml (¼ teaspoon) fennel seeds
- 1 egg
- Sea salt
- Freshly ground pepper to taste

For the hash (all ingredients to be chopped should be about the same size):

- 4 paleo-approved bacon strip, diced
- 4 breakfast sausages, homemade or paleo approved, diced

- 4 eggs
- 1 tablespoons olive oil (optional)
- 1 yellow onion, diced
- 1 green bell pepper, diced
- 1 red bell pepper, diced
- 2 celery stalks, diced
- 1 sweet potato, diced
- 1 zucchini, diced
- 2 garlic cloves, minced
- 1 tablespoon jalapeños pepper, minced
- Sea salt
- fresh ground pepper to taste

INSTRUCTIONS:

Pre-heat the oven at 200ºC/400 F.

For the sausage patties:

1) Place all the ingredients in a mixing bowl and combine well. Let rest and cover with a plastic wrap for at least 30 minutes. Form equal sized patties.

2) In a large frying pan heat some olive oil on high heat. Fry the patties until well done, about 3-4 minutes on each side on medium-high heat. Do not press down too much on the patties while cooking or they will harden.

For the hash:

1) In a large skillet, cook the bacon on high heat for 2-3 minutes until golden. Add onions and garlic, and continue cooking on medium heat for 2-3 minutes. Add sweet potatoes, cook for 5-6 minutes until the bacon is cooked. Add remaining ingredients. Cook for an additional 5-6 minutes

or until all the vegetables are tender crisp. Season with salt and pepper to taste. Remove the pan from heat and reserve.

2) In another frying pan, cook the eggs sunny side up until done. Season with salt and pepper to taste.

3) Spoon ¼ of the hash on a plate, top with one sunny egg. Repeat for each serving.

Nutritional Information (per serving)

Calories: 444

Fat total: 40.1g

Saturated fat: 14.7g

Carbohydrates: 13.3g

Dietary fiber: 5.6g

Sugars: 4.1g

Protein: 14.2g

7. SWEET, GLORIOUS MORNING SMOOTHIE

Serves: 2

Prep Time: 10 minutes

Cooking Time: 0 minutes

INGREDIENTS:

- 500 ml (2 cups) almond milk
- 1 orange, preferably without seeds, peeled and sectioned
- 1 grapefruit, medium size, peeled and sectioned
- 375 ml (1½ cup) frozen mango pieces
- 1 tablespoon of raw honey (optional)

INSTRUCTIONS:

1) Place all the ingredients, except the ice, in a blender. Include the raw honey, if you like it sweeter. Blend until smooth. If it is too liquid-y, add ice cubes and pulse blend until desired consistency.

Nutritional Information (per serving)

Calories: 444

Fat total: 40.1g

Saturated fat: 14.7g

Carbohydrates: 13.3g

Dietary fiber: 5.6g

Sugars: 4.1g

Protein: 14.2g

8. DELICIOUS PALEO WAFFLES

Serves: 4

Prep Time: 15 minutes

Cooking Time: 15 minutes

INGREDIENTS:

- 1 cup almond flour
- 30 ml (2 tablespoons) coconut flour
- ½ teaspoon baking soda
- ¼ teaspoon cinnamon
- ¼ teaspoon salt
- 4 eggs (separated)
- 15 ml (1 tablespoon) olive oil
- ¼ cup coconut milk
- ¼ cup unsweetened organic applesauce or mashed ripe banana (depends on your taste)
- 1 teaspoon vanilla
- Fresh fruits for garnish or unsweetened organic applesauce or maple syrup

INSTRUCTIONS:

1) Lightly grease the waffle maker with coconut butter and

preheat.

2) In a bowl, beat egg whites on high speed for about 3 minutes, until they form stiff peaks.

3) In a bowl, mix flour, baking soda, cinnamon, and salt. In another bowl, whisk egg yolks, milk, applesauce or mashed banana, vanilla, and oil.

4) Add flour mixture to the wet mixture and combine well. Fold in ¼ of the egg whites and mix well. Add another ¼ of egg whites, and gently fold it into the batter. Repeat twice. You should have a light and fluffy batter.

5) Place ⅓ cup to ½ cup of the batter in the greased waffle iron. Close gently and cook until golden browned.

6) Top with fresh fruits or unsweetened organic applesauce or a maple syrup drizzle

Nutritional Information (per serving)

Calories: 444

Fat total: 40.1g

Saturated fat: 14.7g

Carbohydrates: 13.3g

Dietary fiber: 5.6g

Sugars: 4.1g

Protein: 14.2g

9. YUMMY HUNGRY MAN STEAK AND BACON HASH

Serves: 4

Prep Time: 30 minutes

Cooking Time: 25 minutes

INGREDIENTS:

- 4 paleo-approved bacon strips, chopped
- ½ pound of thinly sliced beef strips such as sirloin, chopped
- 4 eggs
- 1 tablespoons olive oil (optional)
- ½ cup chopped onions
- ½ cup green bell pepper, chopped
- ½ cup red bell pepper, chopped
- 1 sweet potato, cubed
- 1 zucchini, cubed
- 2 garlic cloves, minced
- 1 tablespoon jalapeños pepper, minced
- Sea salt & fresh ground pepper to taste

INSTRUCTIONS:

1) Pre-heat the oven at 200ºC/400 F.

2) In a large frying pan, cook the bacon for 2-3 minutes until golden on high heat. Add onions and garlic, and continue cooking on medium heat for 2-3 minutes.

3) Add the beef and sweet potatoes, cook for 5-6 minutes until the meat is cooked. Add remaining ingredients and cook for an additional 10 minutes, or until all the vegetables are tender. Season with salt and pepper to taste. Remove the pan from heat.

4) In another frying pan, cook the eggs sunny side up until done. Season with salt and pepper to taste

5) Spoon ¼ of the meat and vegetables mix on a plate, top with one sunny egg.

6) Repeat for each serving.

Nutritional Information (per serving)

Calories: 444

Fat total: 40.1g

Saturated fat: 14.7g,

Carbohydrates: 13.3g

Dietary fiber: 5.6g

Sugars: 4.1g

Protein: 14.2g

10. NO-CRUST MINI BACON QUICHES

Serves: 8

Prep Time: 15 minutes

Cooking Time: 25 minutes

INGREDIENTS:

- 4 paleo-approved bacon strips, chopped
- 6 eggs
- 2 tablespoons olive oil (optional)
- ½ cup chopped onions
- ½ cup green bell pepper, chopped
- ½ cup red bell pepper, chopped
- Sea salt & fresh ground pepper to taste
- Coconut butter or olive oil for greasing
- Paprika to sprinkle

INSTRUCTIONS:

1) Pre-heat the oven at 190ºC/375ºF.

2) In a large frying pan, cook the bacon for 5 minutes until golden brown on medium-high heat. Add onions, cooking on medium heat for 2 minutes. Add peppers, cook for 2 minutes, season with salt and pepper to taste. Remove the

pan from heat and let cool a few minutes.

3) In the meantime, whisk the eggs vigorously for 2-3 minutes until very fluffy, then add the vegetables and bacon to the eggs and combine well. Season with salt and pepper to taste.

4) Grease generously a muffin pan with olive oil or coconut butter. Fill ¾ of each muffin hole with the egg mixture.

5) Bake the egg muffins in the pre-heated oven for 10-12 minutes or until golden brown. Let cool for 5-10 minutes before unmolding, sprinkle with paprika. Serve hot with slices of tomatoes.

Nutritional Information (per serving)

Calories: 444

Fat total: 40.1g

Saturated fat: 14.7g

Carbohydrates: 13.3g

Dietary fiber: 5.6g

Sugars: 4.1g

Protein: 14.2g

LUNCH RECIPES

11. YUMMY CHICKEN & SPINACH

Serves: 2

Prep Time: 10 minutes

Cooking Time: 15 minutes

INGREDIENTS:

- 45 ml (3 tablespoons) coconut oil
- 1 skinless and boneless chicken breast, cut into strips
- 1 garlic clove, minced
- 1 onion, chopped
- 250 ml (1 cup) spinach, washed and chopped
- Salt & freshly ground black pepper to taste
- 125 ml (½ cup) organic, unsweetened, shredded coconut

INSTRUCTIONS:

1) Heat oil in a large frying pan.

2) Stir in chicken and garlic, and cook for 8 to 10 minutes until a little browned.

3) Add onion and spinach, and continue to cook for 5 minutes until the vegetables are tender.

4) Season with salt and pepper. Sprinkle with coconut and serve.

Nutritional Information (per serving)

Calories: 334

Fat total: 28.6g

Saturated fat: 23.8g

Carbohydrates: 9.0g

Dietary fiber: 3.3g

Sugars: 3.5g

Protein: 13.8g

12. DELIGHTFUL VEGETABLE MEDLEY SOUP

Serves: 2

Prep Time: 15 minutes

Cooking Time: 35 minutes

INGREDIENTS:

- 30 ml (2 tablespoons) coconut oil
- 1 onion, diced
- 2 garlic cloves, chopped
- 5 ml (1 teaspoon) ginger, chopped
- 125 ml (½ cup) cauliflower, chopped
- 125 ml (½ cup) yellow squash, cubed
- 30 ml (2 tablespoons) celery, chopped
- 750 ml (3 cups) vegetable broth
- Salt and pepper to taste
- 15 ml (1 tablespoon) lemon juice

INSTRUCTIONS:

1) Heat oil in a large pan over medium heat.

2) Sauté onion, garlic, and ginger for a few minutes or until

tender and fragrant.

3) Add cauliflower, yellow squash, and celery, and cook for 5 minutes, stirring occasionally.

4) Add broth and bring to a boil on high heat. Bring heat down to medium, cover and cook for 15 to 20 minutes or until vegetables are tender. Remove from heat and cool a little.

5) Place soup in a food processor, and pulse until smooth and thick.

6) Return to soup pan, season, and let soup simmer for 5 minutes until reheated.

7) Ladle soup into a soup bowl, drizzle with lemon juice, and serve.

Nutritional Information (per serving)

Calories: 223

Fat: 15.9g

Saturated fat: 12.4g

Carbohydrates: 11.7g

Dietary fiber: 2.6g

Sugars: 4.6g

Protein: 0.4g

13. TANTALIZING PALEO PRAWNS WITH TOMATO SAUCE

Serves: 2

Prep Time: 5 minutes

Cooking Time: 10 minutes

INGREDIENTS:

- 30 ml (2 tablespoons) olive oil
- 1 red onion, chopped
- 1 cloves garlic, minced
- 225 g (½ pound) prawns
- 2 medium tomatoes, chopped
- 2.5 ml (½ teaspoon) cayenne pepper
- 5 ml (1 teaspoon) oregano
- 30 ml (2 tablespoons) celery, chopped
- 30 ml (2 tablespoons) capers
- 2.5 ml (½ teaspoon) sea salt
- 2.5 ml (½ teaspoon) black pepper

INSTRUCTIONS:

1) Heat oil in a large frying pan.

2) Stir in onion and garlic, and cook for few minutes until fragrant and tender.

3) Add prawns and tomatoes, and cook for 6-7 minutes until prawns are tender.

4) Sprinkle with cayenne pepper, oregano, celery, and capers. Season with salt and pepper and serve.

Nutritional Information (per serving)

Calories: 309

Fat: 16.4g

Saturated fat: 2.7g

Carbohydrates: 13.7g

Dietary fiber: 3.6g

Sugars: 5.7g

Protein: 28.0g

14. FRESH CUCUMBER & WATERMELON SALAD

Serves: 2

Prep Time: 5 minutes

Cooking Time: 0 minutes

INGREDIENTS:

- 1 cucumber, diced
- 1 l (4 cups) watermelon, seeded and diced
- 15 ml (1 tablespoon) red onion, sliced thinly
- 60 ml (4 tablespoons) fresh mint leaves, minced
- 30 ml (2 tablespoons) balsamic vinegar
- 45 ml (3 tablespoons) coconut oil
- Salt & freshly ground black pepper (to taste)
- 30 ml (2 tablespoons) walnuts, chopped

INSTRUCTIONS:

1) Toss all ingredients in a mixing bowl, and season with salt and pepper.

2) Sprinkle with walnuts and serve.

Nutritional Information (per serving)

Calories: 302

Fat total: 25.5g

Saturated fat: 17.9g

Carbohydrates: 19.3g

Dietary fiber: 2.8g

Sugars: 9.8g

Protein: 4.2g

15. CREAMY MUSHROOM CREAM SOUP

Serves: 3

Prep Time: 10 minutes

Cooking Time: 20 minutes

INGREDIENTS:

- 30 ml (2 tablespoons) coconut oil
- 1 onion, chopped
- 1 garlic clove, minced
- 2 avocados, sliced
- 250 ml (1 cup) mushrooms, sliced
- 1 red sweet pepper, chopped
- 2 tomatoes, sliced
- 4 sprigs basil leaves
- 750 ml (3 cups) chicken stock
- 250 ml (1 cup) coconut cream
- Salt & freshly ground black pepper to taste

INSTRUCTIONS:

1) Heat oil in a pan.

2) Add onion and garlic, and cook for 3 to 4 minutes until tender.

3) Add avocado, mushrooms, red sweet pepper, tomatoes, and basil leaves, and continue to cook until the vegetables are tender.

4) Add water and bring to a boil. Cover and cook for 15 minutes.

5) Sprinkle with salt and pepper.

6) When cooked, cool a little, place soup into food processor, and blend until smooth and creamy.

7) Reheat, ladle in a soup bowl, and serve.

Nutritional Information (per serving)

Calories: 389

Fat total: 35.6g

Saturated fat: 10.7g

Carbohydrates: 20.8g

Dietary fiber: 11.9g

Sugars: 15.6g

Protein: 14.1g

16. SMOOTH BROCCOLI & PINE NUTS SOUP

Serves: 2

Prep Time: 5 minutes

Cooking Time: 30 minutes

INGREDIENTS:

- 30 ml (2 tablespoons) coconut oil
- 1 onion, diced
- 1 l (4 cups) broccoli
- 750 ml (3 cups) vegetable broth
- 60 ml (¼ cup) pine-nuts

INSTRUCTIONS:

1) Heat oil in a large pan.

2) Stir in onion and broccoli, cook for few minutes until broccoli is a little tender.

3) Add broth and pine nuts and bring to a boil. Cover and cook on medium low for 10 to 15 minutes.

4) Place soup in a food processor and pulse until smooth and thick.

5) Return to soup pan and let it simmer for 5 minutes.

6) Ladle soup into a serving bowl and serve hot.

Nutritional Information (per serving)

Calories: 312

Fat total: 22.4g

Saturated fat: 12.8g

Carbohydrates: 14.1g

Dietary fiber: 3.9g

Sugars: 5.2g

Protein: 13.8g

17. SPICY BRUSSEL SPROUTS & BACON WITH TANDOORI DRUMSTICKS

Serves: 4

Prep Time: 15 minutes

Cooking Time: 25 minutes

INGREDIENTS:

- 15 ml (1 tablespoon) olive oil
- 2 slices paleo-approved bacon, diced
- 500 ml (2 cups) brussel sprouts, trimmed and halved
- 1 onion, sliced
- 10 ml (2 teaspoons) freshly squeezed lemon juice
- Salt and freshly ground pepper to taste

INSTRUCTIONS:

1) Heat oil in a pan over medium heat.

2) Stir in bacon and cook for 4-5 minutes until bacon is a little browned, add onions and sauté for 2-3 minutes.

3) Add brussel sprouts continue to cook for 15 more minutes,

stirring occasionally, until sprouts are tender.

4) Drizzle lemon juice, season with salt and pepper.

5) Serve with leftover tandoori chicken drumsticks.

Nutritional Information (per serving – Brussels sprouts only)

Calories: 224

Fat total: 15.1g

Saturated fat: 3.7g

Carbohydrates: 9.3g

Dietary fiber: 2.8g

Sugars: 3.2g

Protein: 9.1g

18. CRUNCHY SALMON & ASPARAGUS SALAD

Serves: 2

Prep Time: 10 minutes

Cooking Time: 5 minutes

INGREDIENTS:

- 250 ml (1 cup) salmon, boiled and shredded
- 125 ml (½ cup) onion, chopped
- 125 ml (½ cup) celery, chopped
- 125 ml (½ cup) asparagus
- 125 ml (½ cup) cherry tomatoes, halved
- 30 ml (2 tablespoons) olive oil
- Spring mix salad
- Salt & pepper to taste

INSTRUCTIONS:

1) Steam asparagus in boiling water for 5-6 minutes. Drain asparagus and immediately add to a bowl filled with cold water to stop cooking process.

2) Toss all ingredients in a mixing bowl and season with salt and pepper.

3) Serve on a bed of spring mix salad.

Nutritional Information (per serving)

Calories: 267

Fat total: 19.6g

Saturated fat: 2.8g

Carbohydrates: 6.3g

Dietary fiber: 2.2g

Sugars: 3.3g

Protein: 18.8g

19. CREAMY SAUTÉED LEEKS WITH SALMON

Serves: 2

Prep Time: 10 minutes

Cooking Time: 30 minutes

INGREDIENTS:

- 30 ml (2 tablespoons) almond butter, separated
- 125 ml (½ cup) leeks, chopped
- 30 ml (2 tablespoons) celery, chopped
- 2 carrots, sliced
- 2 salmon fillets, cut into strips
- 30 ml (2 tablespoons) lemon juice
- Salt & pepper to taste

INSTRUCTIONS:

1) Melt half of the almond butter in a sauté pan over medium.

2) Stir in carrots, and cook for 5 minutes, stirring often. Add leeks and celery, and continue cooking for 5 minutes more or until carrots are crisply tender. Remove vegetables onto a plate, and set aside.

3) Heat remaining butter in the same pan, and add salmon. Let simmer, stirring occasionally, for 15 minutes until fish

is cooked through. Add in sautéed vegetables, and stir for 2 minutes until vegetables are heated through.

4) Drizzle lemon juice, season with salt and pepper and serve.

Nutritional Information (per serving)

Calories: 380

Fat total: 20.4g

Saturated fat: 2.6g

Carbohydrates: 12.3g

Dietary fiber: 2.9g

Sugars: 4.2g

Protein: 39.0g

20. SWEET AND SOUR LEMON GRILLED CHICKEN

Serves: 2

Prep Time: 5 minutes

Cooking Time: 25 minutes

INGREDIENTS:

- 2 chicken thighs
- 30 ml (2 tablespoons) coconut oil
- Pinch of salt and freshly ground black pepper
- 30 ml (2 teaspoons) lemon juice
- ½ tablespoon lemon zest

INSTRUCTIONS:

1) Preheat a grill pan to high.

2) Toss chicken in a bowl with oil, and sprinkle with salt and pepper.

3) Place chicken on grill pan over medium.

4) Grill thighs for 10 minutes on each side, turning occasionally (every 2-3 minutes), until thighs are cooked through. Then bring heat to high, and grill for 4 minutes on both sides to obtain visible grill marks.

5) Serve on a platter drizzled with lemon juice and sprinkled with lemon zest.

Nutritional Information (per serving)

Calories: 385

Fat total: 24.0g

Saturated fat: 14.6g

Carbohydrates: 0.7g

Dietary fiber: 0.0g

Sugars: 0.0g

Protein: 40.6g

21. COLOURFUL SALMON SALAD

Serves: 2

Prep Time: 15 minutes

Cooking Time: 0 minute

INGREDIENTS:

- 250 ml (1 cup) salmon, steamed until done, shredded
- 2 cucumbers, peeled and chopped
- 1 onion, chopped
- 1 large tomato, diced
- 1 avocado, chopped
- 30 ml (2 tablespoons) olive oil
- 30 ml (2 tablespoons) lemon juice
- 30 ml (2 tablespoons) fresh dill
- 125 ml (½ cup) lettuce leaves, shredded
- Pinch of salt and freshly ground black pepper

INSTRUCTIONS:

1) Toss and combine well all ingredients in a salad bowl. Season with salt and pepper.

2) Serve and enjoy.

Nutritional Information (per serving)

Calories: 300

Fat total: 24.1g

Saturated fat: 3.0g

Carbohydrates: 14.9g

Dietary fiber: 7.4g

Sugars: 3.9g

Protein: 7.7g

22. DELICIOUS STUFFED SEA BASS

Serves: 4

Prep Time: 15 minutes

Cooking Time: 25 minutes

INGREDIENTS:

- 4 sea bass about 350 to 450 grams (¾ to 1 pound) each, cleaned, head removed

- 125 ml (½ cup) olive oil

- 45 ml (3 tablespoons) olive oil

- 225 g (½ pound) white mushrooms, sliced

- 1 tablespoon fresh parsley, minced

- 1 green pepper, diced

- Freshly squeezed lemon juice to taste

- Sea salt & fresh ground pepper to taste

INSTRUCTIONS:

1) Pre-heat the oven at 215ºC/425ºF.

2) Salt and pepper the inside of the bass. Add lemon juice to taste.

3) Place each fish on a foil sheet large enough to cover the fish.

4) Melt half of the butter in a medium size frying pan, add the

shallots, and cook 2-3 minutes. Add the mushroom, pepper, and parsley. Season with salt and pepper to taste, and cook for an additional 6 minutes until vegetables are tender.

5)   Stuff each fish with ¼ of the vegetable mix, and brush the fish with olive oil. Seal the aluminum foil well. Place the foil packets on a baking sheet. Cook for 16 minutes.

6) Take out of the oven and make sure the fish is well cooked. If not, bake for an additional 2 minutes or until cooked.

7)   Serve with lemon slices and your favorite vegetables.

Nutritional Information (per serving)

Calories: 444

Fat total: 40.1g

Saturated fat: 14.7g

Carbohydrates: 13.3g

Dietary fiber: 5.6g

Sugars: 4.1g

Protein: 14.2g

23. TASTY PALEO SAUSAGE DELIGHT

Serves: 4

Prep Time: 15 minutes

Cooking Time: 25 minutes

INGREDIENTS:

- 6 paleo-approved sausages of your choice
- 60 ml (¼ cup) olive oil
- 60 ml (¼ cup) apple cider vinegar
- 20 white mushrooms, trimmed
- ¼ cup fresh flat parsley, minced
- 2 sweet peppers, sliced in 1 inch strips
- 2 red onions, sliced in ½ inch strips
- Sea salt & fresh ground pepper to taste

INSTRUCTIONS:

1) Pre-heat the oven at 200ºC/400°F.

2) In a large mixing bowl, combine all ingredients except parsley. Season with salt and freshly ground pepper to taste.

3) Lay the sausages and vegetables mix on a parchment paper-covered baking sheet, and cook for 40 minutes.

4) Sprinkle with parsley and serve with your favorite mustard

and a side of slaw.

Nutritional Information (per serving)

Calories: 444

Fat total: 40.1g

Saturated fat: 14.7g

Carbohydrates: 13.3g

Dietary fiber: 5.6g

Sugars: 4.1g

Protein: 14.2g

24. TANTALIZING ROASTED BEEF WITH NUTTY VEGETABLES

Serves: 4

Prep Time: 15 minutes

Cooking Time: 35 minutes

INGREDIENTS:

- 30 ml (2 tablespoons) olive oil
- 450 g (2 pounds) lean beef steak brisket, sliced
- 30 ml (2 tablespoons) grainy Dijon Mustard
- Montreal steak spice to taste
- Garlic powder to taste
- 1 onion, sliced
- 15 ml (1 tablespoon) garlic, minced
- 250 ml (1 cup) asparagus, sliced
- 2 zucchinis, cubed
- 30 ml (2 tablespoons) almond butter
- 30 ml (2 tablespoons) almond slivers (optional)
- Salt and pepper to taste

INSTRUCTIONS:

1) Preheat the oven to 160ºC/325°F.

2) Heat oil in a skillet on high heat.

3) Rub each steak with mustard, Montreal steak spices, and garlic. When the skillet is hot, stir in the steak slices, and cook for 1-2 minutes on each side until beef is nicely colored.

4) Transfer beef to a baking dish, season with salt and pepper. Place in preheated oven and bake for 10-15 minutes, depending on steak thickness and how you like your steak cooked. When the steaks are cooked to your liking, remove from oven and let rest for a few minutes before serving. This will make your steak juicier.

5) While steaks are baking, in the same skillet, add some more olive oil if necessary, sauté onions and almond slivers (optional) for 2-3 minutes, stirring often. Add asparagus and zucchini and cook 4-5 minutes until vegetables are tender but still crispy. Remove from heat, add almond butter and parsley. Set aside.

6) Serve each steak with a generous portion of the nutty vegetables.

Nutritional Information (per serving)

Calories: 449

Fat total: 29.0g

Saturated fat: 7.8g

Carbohydrates: 9.5g

Dietary fiber: 2.5g

Sugars: 3.9g

Protein: 37.5g

25. OILY PORK CHOPS WITH APPLE

Serves: 2

Prep Time: 10 minutes

Cooking Time: 20 minutes

INGREDIENTS:

- 15 ml (1 tablespoon) coconut oil
- 2 pork chops
- 1 large onion, sliced
- 2 apples, sliced
- Salt & freshly ground black pepper to taste

INSTRUCTIONS:

1) Heat oil in a large pan.
2) Put chops in the pan, and cook for 5 minutes on each side until golden brown.
3) Add onion and apples, and continue to cook for 7 to 9 minutes until the onion and apples are tender.
4) Sprinkle with salt and pepper and serve.

Nutritional Information (per serving)

Calories: 439

Fat total: 26.7g

Saturated fat: 13.3g

Carbohydrates: 31.9g

Dietary fiber: 5.9g

Sugars: 21.9g

Protein: 18.7g

DINNER RECIPES

26. FLESHY TILAPIA WITH THAI CURRY

Serves: 2

Prep Time: 10 minutes

Cooking Time: 25 minutes

INGREDIENTS:

- 125 ml (½ cup) coconut milk
- 250 ml (1 cup) fresh basil leaves
- 60 ml (4 tablespoons) Thai curry paste
- 30 ml (2 tablespoons) olive oil
- 2 tilapia fillets
- 1 large red bell pepper, deseeded, julienne
- 1 onion, sliced
- 60 ml (¼ cup) scallions, sliced
- 30 ml (2 tablespoons) fish sauce
- Salt & freshly ground black pepper to taste

INSTRUCTIONS:

1) Place coconut milk, basil leaves, and Thai curry paste into food processor and blend until smooth.

2) Heat oil in a large pan. Add tilapia fillets, and cook for 5 minutes on each side until a little browned. Remove tilapia

to a plate, and set aside.

3) Add red bell peppers, onion, and scallions in the same pan, and cook until the vegetables are tender.

4) Add coconut milk mixture, and cook for 5 minutes until it thickens. Add in reserved fish fillets; simmer until tilapia is heated through.

5) Drizzle fish sauce, season with salt and pepper and serve.

Nutritional Information (per serving)

Calories: 441

Fat total: 29.7g

Saturated fat: 15.1g

Carbohydrates: 21.1g

Dietary fiber: 4.7g

Sugars: 10.6g

Protein: 25.3g

27. YUMMY PIRI PIRI CHICKEN

Serves: 4

Prep Time: 30 minutes

Cooking Time: 65 minutes

Marinade time: 4 hr up to 12 hr

INGREDIENTS:

- 2 whole organic chicken
- 1 tablespoon of Piri Piri spice mix
- 4 garlic cloves, minced
- 1 onion
- 60 ml (¼ cup) freshly squeezed lemon juice
- 60 ml (¼cup) organic maple syrup
- 5 ml (1 teaspoon) sea salt
- 85 ml (⅓ cup) olive oil
- 30 ml (2 tablespoons) apple cider vinegar
- Sea salt and fresh ground pepper to taste

INSTRUCTIONS:

1) Mix all the ingredients except the chickens in a food processor. Blend until you obtain a smooth marinade.

2) Place the chicken on a working surface, breast side down. With a large and sharp knife, cut open the back of the chicken so that it will flatten and open up. Turn the chicken over, and press firmly to flatten. Repeat for the second chicken.

3) In a large zip lock bag, place one chicken in with half of the marinade. Repeat with the second chicken. Refrigerate for a minimum of 4 hours and up to 12 hours.

4) Remove both chicken from the marinade, and place in a roasting oven pan. Place the chickens, breast side facing up. Season with salt and pepper to taste. Reserve the marinade.

5) Place the excess marinade in a small sauce pan, and cook on low heat for 20 minutes

6) Place the chickens on the middle rack, in preheated 400°F oven, and cook for 30 minutes.

7) After 30 minutes, take out the chicken, smear with some of the marinade on both sides, and cook for another 30 minutes.

8) Brush the breast side with the rest of the marinade, and broil for 5 minutes.

9) Cut the chicken in pieces, and serve with steamed vegetables of your choice.

Nutritional Information (per serving)

Calories: 444

Fat total: 40.1g

Saturated fat: 14.7g

Carbohydrates: 13.3g

Dietary fiber: 5.6g

Sugars: 4.1g

Protein: 14.2g

28. FLESHY NUTTY TILAPIA FILLETS

Serves: 4

Prep Time: 15 minutes

Cooking Time: 10 minutes

INGREDIENTS:

- 4 large Tilapia fillets
- 15 ml (1 tablespoon) black peppercorn
- 8 ml (½ tablespoon) fennel seeds
- 8 ml (½ tablespoon) smoked paprika
- 45 ml (3 tablespoons) coconut butter or grass fed butter
- 125 ml (½ cup) of pecan
- 15 ml (1 tablespoon) fresh flat leaf parsley, chopped
- Sea salt & fresh ground pepper to taste
- 1 lemon, sliced

INSTRUCTIONS:

1) Using a pestle and mortar, crush and grind together peppercorn, fennel seeds, and paprika

2) Season both sides of the tilapia with the spices.

3) Using a frying pan, melt 2 tablespoons of the butter on medium heat. Add the fillets, and cook for 4 minutes, turn

the tilapia over and cook for an additional 3 to 4 minutes until the fish is done.

4) Place your cooked fillets on a warm serving plate, and reserve.

5) In the same hot frying pan, add the rest of the butter and the pecans. Cook for about 1 minute. Add some lemon juice to taste, and mix well.

6) Place the lemony nuts on the fillets, sprinkle with the parsley, and serve with your favorite side vegetables and lemon slices.

Nutritional Information (per serving)

Calories: 444

Fat total: 40.1g

Saturated fat: 14.7g

Carbohydrates: 13.3g

Dietary fiber: 5.6g

Sugars: 4.1g

Protein: 14.2g

29. DELIGHTFUL TANDOORI CHICKEN DRUMSTICKS & MANGO CHUTNEY

Serves: 8

Prep Time: 45 minutes

Cooking Time: 30 minutes

Marinade time: 4 hr or more

INGREDIENTS:

- 16 chicken drumsticks
- Tandoori mix:
- 250 ml (1 cup) coconut milk
- Juice of 2 lemons
- 125 ml (½ cup) olive oil
- 60ml (¼ cup) tandoori spices
- 15 ml (1 tablespoon) red sweet paprika
- Sea salt & fresh ground pepper to taste

Mango Chutney:

- 30 ml (2 tablespoons) olive oil

- 2 garlic cloves, minced
- 15 ml (1 tablespoon) fresh ginger, minced
- 2 mango, peeled and cubed
- 30 ml (2 tablespoons) raw honey
- 60 ml (¼ cup) white vinegar
- 60 ml (¼ cup) water
- 2 cinnamon sticks
- 4 cloves
- 1-2 pinches of crushed chilies to taste
- Sea salt & fresh ground pepper to taste

INSTRUCTIONS:

1) Put all the ingredients for the tandoori mix together in a ziplock bag or a container, place the chicken in, and let marinate for at least 4 hr.

2) For the chutney, in a small frying pan, heat the oil on high, reduce heat to medium, and cook the garlic and ginger for 2 to 3 minutes. Add all the remaining ingredients and cook covered for an additional 15 minutes on low heat. Remove the cover and cook another 10 minutes, or until you obtain a consistent chutney. Cool before serving

3) Preheat oven to 400°F.

4) Place the drumsticks on a slightly oiled baking sheet. Cook for 30 minutes until the chicken is well cooked.

5) Serve with the mango chutney and your favorite steamed vegetables.

Nutritional Information (per serving)

Calories: 444

Fat total: 40.1g

Saturated fat: 14.7g

Carbohydrates: 13.3g

Dietary fiber: 5.6 g

Sugars: 4.1g

Protein: 14.2g

30. DELICIOUS PALEO ORANGE CHICKEN

Serves: 2

Prep Time: 5 minutes

Cooking Time: 20 minutes

INGREDIENTS:

- 15 ml (1 tablespoon) coconut oil
- 225 g (½ pound) boneless chicken breast, cut into strips
- 1 garlic clove, minced
- 125 ml (½ cup) fresh orange juice
- 30 ml (2 tablespoons) grated orange
- Salt & pepper for seasoning

INSTRUCTIONS:

1) Heat oil in a large frying pan over medium heat.

2) Stir in garlic and sauté 1 minute. Add chicken strips and cook a few minutes, stirring occasionally until chicken is not pink any more.

3) Add orange juice, cover, and continue to cook for 15 minutes over medium-low, until chicken is tender and juices almost run clear.

4) Sprinkle grated orange, season with salt and pepper, and

serve.

Nutritional Information (per serving)

Calories: 310

Fat total: 15.3g

Saturated fat: 8.2g

Carbohydrates: 8.3g

Dietary fiber: 0.0g

Sugars: 6.3g

Protein: 33.5g

31. YUMMY BEEF GOULASH

Serves: 4

Prep Time: 20 minutes

Cooking Time: 2 hr

INGREDIENTS:

- 1 kg (2 pounds) boneless stew beef, such as chuck roast
- 30 ml (2 tablespoons) olive oil
- 1 large onion, chopped
- 4 garlic clove, minced
- 5 ml (1 teaspoon) caraway seeds
- 1 red bell pepper, deseeded, julienne
- 2 sweet potatoes, peeled and cubed
- 2 tomatoes, chopped
- 5 ml (1 teaspoon) salt
- 15 ml (1 tablespoon) jalapeños pepper, minced
- 500 ml (2 cups) beef broth
- Salt & pepper

INSTRUCTIONS:

1) Cut beef into same size cube, about 4-5 cm (1-2 inches). Dry

beef with paper towel.

2) Heat oil in a large and deep skillet. Add beef and brown the meat very well, in batches if necessary. For proper browning, the beef cubes should not touch each other in the pan. Remove the meat from the skillet and reserve.

3) Add oil if necessary. Sauté onions for few minutes until translucent. Add in garlic, and cook for 2 minutes. Add the spices, mix well. Add red bell peppers and tomatoes and cook for 5 minutes. Add the reserved beef.

4) Season with salt and pepper to taste, and add the jalapeños chili.

5) Add broth, and bring to a boil on high heat. Reduce heat to medium-low. Cover and cook for 1 hr. Add sweet potatoes, and cook for an additional 30 minutes. The meat should be very tender and easily cut with a fork. Taste and adjust seasoning with salt or pepper.

6) Serve hot with a side green salad.

Nutritional Information (per serving)

Calories: 269

Fat total: 23.7g

Saturated fat: 7.5g

Carbohydrates: 6.6g

Dietary fiber: 1.6g

Sugars: 3.3g

Protein: 7.9g

32. BAKED BEEF WITH VEGETABLES

Serves: 4

Prep Time: 10 minutes

Marinating Time: 2 hours

Cooking Time: 35 minutes

INGREDIENTS:

- 30 ml (2 tablespoons) coconut oil
- 225 g (½ pound) boneless beef strips
- 1 small red onion, chopped
- 2 cloves garlic, chopped
- 125 ml (½ cup) carrots, sliced
- 1 l (4 cups) butternut squash, chopped
- 1 sweet potato, chopped
- 2.5 ml (½ teaspoon) dried thyme
- 2.5 ml (½ teaspoon) dried rosemary
- 60 ml (¼ cup) coconut amino
- 2.5 ml (½ teaspoon) ground black pepper

INSTRUCTIONS:

1)   In a large bowl, add all ingredients except vegetables. Mix

well. Let marinate for 30 minutes.

2) Preheat the oven to 180ºC/350°F.

3) Toss in vegetables as well.

4) Place beef and vegetables in the baking dish, cover the dish completely with foil, and bake for 30 to 35 minutes. After that, remove foil, and roast again for 10 minutes.

Nutritional Information (per serving)

Calories: 353

Fat total: 27.6g

Saturated fat: 14.9g

Carbohydrates: 17.8g

Dietary fiber: 3.3g

Sugars: 4.8g

Protein: 9.8g

33. BEAUTIFUL HERB-CRUSTED PORK TENDERLOIN

Serves: 4

Prep Time: 15 minutes

Marinating Time: 2 hr

Cooking Time: 40 minutes

INGREDIENTS:

- 2 pork tenderloins (about 350 to 450 g (¾ to 1 pound) each)
- 2 cloves garlic, minced
- 45 ml (3 tablespoons) fresh rosemary
- 45 ml (3 tablespoons) fresh thyme
- 15 ml (1 tablespoon) smoked paprika
- ½ onion, cut in a few pieces
- 5 ml (1 teaspoon) sea salt
- 5 ml (1 teaspoon) ground black pepper
- 60 ml (¼ cup) freshly squeezed lime juice

INSTRUCTIONS:

1) Preheat the oven to 180ºC/350°F.

2) In a food processor, add all ingredients except pork. Pulse until it becomes a smooth paste.

3) In a bowl, add pork and herb mixture. Mix until well combined. Cover and refrigerate for 2 hours to marinate.

4) Place pork into baking dish. Bake for 30 to 40 minutes until pork is fully cooked.

5) Cut into slices before serving.

6) Serve with a medley of steamed vegetables and unsweetened organic applesauce if desired.

Nutritional Information (per serving)

Calories: 165

Fat total: 5.9g

Saturated fat: 2.3g

Carbohydrates: 9.4g

Dietary fiber: 2.9g

Sugars: 1.1g

Protein: 20.3g

34. TASTY GROUND BEEF WITH KALE

Serves: 2

Prep Time: 10 minutes

Cooking Time: 15 minutes

INGREDIENTS:

- 15 ml (1 tablespoon) coconut oil
- 225 g (½ pound) ground beef
- 2 small red chilies, finely sliced
- 1 large bunch of kale, trimmed and chopped
- 1 lemon
- Salt and pepper for seasoning

INSTRUCTIONS:

1) Heat oil in a large frying pan.
2) Stir in beef and red chilies, cook for few minutes until a little browned.
3) Add kale, and continue to cook until the kale is just wilted.
4) Drizzle lemon juice, season with salt and pepper, and serve.

Nutritional Information (per serving)

Calories: 295

Fat total: 14.2g

Saturated fat: 8.7g

Carbohydrates: 4.7g

Dietary fiber: 0.7g.

Sugars: 0.0g

Protein: 35.9g

DESSERT RECIPES

35. SWEET RASPBERRY ICE CREAM

Serves: 2

Prep Time: 10 minutes

Cooking Time: 0 minutes

INGREDIENTS:

- 250 ml (1 cup) coconut milk
- 60 ml (¼ cup) raw honey
- 125 ml (½ cup) raspberry, pureed
- 5 ml (1 teaspoon) vanilla extract
- 2.5 ml (½ teaspoon) pumpkin pie spice

For garnishing

- 30 ml (2 tablespoons) walnuts, chopped

INSTRUCTIONS:

1) In a bowl, add all ice cream ingredients and mix till well combined. Pour into ice cream maker.

2) Freeze ice cream until fully set.

3) Garnish with walnuts.

Nutritional Information (per serving)

Calories: 191

Fat total: 2.6g

Saturated fat: 2.5g

Carbohydrates: 43.5g

Dietary fiber: 1.9g

Sugars: 6.3g

Protein: 1.2g

36. FRESH BERRIES WITH ALMONDS

Serves: 2

Prep Time: 5 minutes

Cooking Time: 0 minutes

INGREDIENTS:

- 250 ml (1 cup) fresh berries
- 30 ml (2 tablespoons) balsamic vinegar
- 30 ml (2 tablespoons) maple syrup
- 85 ml (⅓ cup) almonds, toasted and chopped

INSTRUCTIONS:

1) Combine all ingredients in a bowl and serve.

Nutritional Information (per serving)

Calories: 181

Fat total: 8.1g

Saturated fat: 0.6g

Carbohydrates: 25.5g

Dietary fiber: 4.5g

Sugars: 17.6g

Protein: 3.8g

37. TASTY CHOCOLATE BARK

Serves: 4

Prep Time: 5 minutes

Cooking Time: 3 minute

Refrigerating Time: 1 hour

INGREDIENTS:

- 125 ml (½ cup) dark chocolate (70% or more cocoa), chopped
- 125 ml (½ cup) dried cherries, chopped
- 250 ml (1 cup) pecans
- 1 ml (¼ teaspoon) fleur de sel or any coarse salt

INSTRUCTIONS:

1) Melt chocolate in a double boiler saucepan on medium low heat, or in the microwave until just melted.

2) Stir in cherries, pecans, and salt, and cook for few seconds.

3) Spread chocolate mixture on a baking dish with a spatula.

4) Refrigerate for at least 1 hour until set.

5) Break into bite size pieces, serve, and enjoy!

Nutritional Information (per serving)

Calories: 221

Fat total: 16.0g

Saturated fat: 5.2g

Carbohydrates: 18.1g

Dietary fiber: 2.1g

Sugars: 11.4g

Protein: 2.9g

38. HONEY COATED WALNUTS & PEACHES

Serves: 2

Prep Time: 5 minutes

Cooking Time: 3 minutes

INGREDIENTS:

- 30 ml (2 tablespoons) almond butter
- 60 ml (4 tablespoons) raw honey
- 2 peaches, sliced
- 60 ml (4 tablespoons) walnuts, chopped
- 5 ml (1 teaspoon) cinnamon, ground

INSTRUCTIONS:

1) Heat butter and honey in a saucepan.

2) Stir in peach and walnuts and cook for 3 minutes.

3) Sprinkle with cinnamon. Serve and enjoy!

Nutritional Information (per serving)

Calories: 367

Fat total: 18.5g

Saturated fat: 1.4g

Carbohydrates: 49.3g

Dietary fiber: 3.8g

Sugars: 42.9g

Protein: 8.2g

39. CRUNCHY ALMOND FLORENTINE

Serves: 2

Prep Time: 10 minutes

Cooking Time: 30 minutes

INGREDIENTS:

- 125 ml (½ cup) almond meal
- 2.5 ml (½ teaspoon) cinnamon
- 30 ml (2 tablespoons) nutmeg
- 2.5 ml (½ teaspoon) vanilla extract
- 45 ml (3 tablespoons) maple syrup
- Pinch of salt

INSTRUCTIONS:

1)   Preheat the oven to 180ºC/350ºF. Lightly grease a baking dish.

2) Combine all ingredients in bowl, and mix well.

3) Put small portions of the dough with a spoon on the baking dish.

4) Bake for 25 to 30 minutes.

Nutritional Information (per serving)

Calories: 256

Fat total: 14.3g

Saturated fat: 2.7g

Carbohydrates: 29.3g

Dietary fiber: 4.7g

Sugars: 20.9g

Protein: 5.5g

40. APPLE PUDDING WITH COCONUT WHIPPED CREAM

Serves: 2

Prep Time: 5 minutes

Cooking Time: 5 minutes

INGREDIENTS:

- 45 ml (3 tablespoons) coconut oil
- 250 ml (1 cup) coconut milk
- 30 ml (2 tablespoons) raw honey
- 2 apples, peeled and sliced
- 5 ml (1 teaspoon) cinnamon
- 125 ml (½ cup) coconut cream
- 5 ml (1 teaspoon) vanilla

INSTRUCTIONS:

1) Heat oil in a large pan.

2) Add coconut milk, honey, and apples. Cook for 5 minutes until apples are tender.

3) Remove from the heat. Let it cool.

4) Place apple mixture in a food processor, and pulse until

smooth.

5)   In a small mixing bowl, add coconut cream and vanilla. With an electric mixer, whip the cream until it form peaks and has a whipped cream texture, about 3 minutes. Add raw honey, and mix in with a spoon

6)   Sprinkle with cinnamon, and serve with the coconut whipped cream.

Nutritional Information (per serving)

Calories: 319

Fat total: 12.1 g

Saturated fat: 10.9

Carbohydrates: 54.5

Dietary fiber: 5.0g

Sugars: 28.6g

Protein: 1.5g

41. SWEET BANANA WITH COCONUT ALMOND BUTTER

Serves: 2

Prep Time: 10 minutes

Cooking Time: 0 minutes

INGREDIENTS:

- 2 bananas, sliced
- 60 ml (4 tablespoons) coconut milk
- 60 ml (4 tablespoons) almond butter
- 0.5 ml (⅛ teaspoon) cinnamon

INSTRUCTIONS:

1) Toss all ingredients in a mixing bowl, and sprinkle with cinnamon.

2) Let it rest 5 minutes before serving in dessert bowls.

Nutritional Information (per serving)

Calories: 378

Fat total: 25.6g

Saturated fat: 8.1g

Carbohydrates: 34.4g

Dietary fiber: 5.0g

Sugars: 15.4g

Protein: 8.8g

42. CREAMY COCONUT WHIPPED CREAM

Serves: 2

Prep Time: 5 minutes

Refrigerating Time: 2-3 hr

INGREDIENTS:

- 250 ml (1 cup) coconut cream
- 250 ml (1 cup) coconut milk
- 1 ml (¼ teaspoon) cinnamon
- 2.5 ml (½ teaspoon) vanilla extract
- 1 ml (¼ teaspoon) ground nutmeg

INSTRUCTIONS:

1) Place all the ingredients in food processor, and blend until smooth and creamy.

2) Pour coconut cream in 4 cups, and refrigerate for at least 2 to 3 hours.

3) Serve and enjoy!

Nutritional Information (per serving)

Calories: 559

Fat total: 57.6g

Saturated fat: 51.0g

Carbohydrates: 14.0g

Dietary fiber: 5.6g

Sugars: 8.4g

Protein: 5.6g

43. SWEET PALEO PUMPKIN MUFFINS

Serves: 5

Prep Time: 2 minutes

Cooking Time: 25 minutes

INGREDIENTS:

- 750 ml (1½ cup) almond flour
- 60 ml (4 tablespoons) coconut flour
- 5 ml (1 teaspoon) baking soda
- 5 ml (1 teaspoon) baking powder
- 2.5 ml (½ teaspoon) pumpkin pie spice
- 2.5 ml (½ teaspoon) ground cinnamon
- 0.5 ml (⅛ teaspoon) sea salt
- 2 large eggs
- ¾ cup pumpkin puree
- 60 ml (¼ cup) raw honey
- 30 ml (2 teaspoons) almond butter
- 15 ml (1 tablespoon) almonds, toasted and chopped

INSTRUCTIONS:

1) Preheat the oven to 200ºC/400°F.

2) Whisk almond flour, coconut flour, baking soda, baking powder, and pumpkin pie spice in a mixing bowl. Sprinkle with cinnamon and salt.

3) In another bowl whisk the eggs. Add pumpkin puree, honey, and butter.

4) Mix wet ingredients with dry ingredients. Fill the batter in muffin cups until each is almost full.

5) Sprinkle with almonds.

6) Bake for 20 to 25 minutes, or until a toothpick inserted in the center comes out clean.

Nutritional Information (per serving)

Calories: 189

Fat total: 8.7g

Saturated fat: 1.4g

Carbohydrates: 23.7

Dietary fiber: 4.5g

Sugars: 16.1g

Protein: 6.3g

44. CREAM BANANA TREAT WITH CRANBERRIES AND COCONUT MILK

Serves: 2

Prep Time: 5 minutes

Cooking Time: 0 minutes

INGREDIENTS:

- 1 large banana, sliced
- 30 ml (2 tablespoons) almond butter
- 30 ml (2 tablespoons) coconut milk
- 125 ml (½ cup) cranberries
- Pinch of cinnamon

INSTRUCTIONS:

1) Combine bananas with almond butter and coconut milk in a large bowl.

2) Add cranberries on top and sprinkle with cinnamon before serving.

Nutritional Information (per serving)

Calories: 208

Fat total: 12.9g

Saturated fat: 4.1g

Carbohydrates: 22.2g

Dietary fiber: 3.9g

Sugars: 9.8g

Protein: 4.6g.

CONCLUSION

I hope that the information shared with you here will positively help you learn all that meal prepping entails. At this moment, you have a better idea of how to live a healthy lifestyle, how to prepare your meals faster, how to avoid mistakes, how to properly store your meals, etc. Also, the recipes provided in the book are paleo recipes, which will eventually help you lose weight.

Remember, perseverance and hard-work lead to success, so don't give up easily; practice, practice, practice. All you need now is to put together all the necessary materials and be ready to embark on this journey. Meal prepping will be quite an adventure, but you will soon find out that the rewards are real and fruitful.

[1] No cooking time

www.ingramcontent.com/pod-product-compliance
Lightning Source LLC
Chambersburg PA
CBHW060109260726
48658CB00004B/1468